THE OBESITY CONCEPT

Overcoming food cravings instant weight loss and reviving your youthful and healthier body

By

Christopher L. Dill

Disclaimer

Table of contents

Introduction

A common health issue, obesity arises when the body stores an excessive amount of fat, usually as a result of lifestyle factors including food preferences and exercise levels. Because of the serious threats this disorder poses to general health, it is critical to comprehend its causes and investigate practical preventive and therapeutic techniques.

Chapter 1

Understanding the obesity epidemic: The causes, the What or how factors and its health effects

Being overweight and obese together structure one of the leading preventable causes of death within the U.S. Obesity may be a chronic disease that will seriously affect your health. To be overweight means you have extra weight, while obesity means you have a high amount of additional body fat. An overweight or obese person could be at risk of health problems.

These include coronary heart conditions, type 2 diabetes, asthma, high cholesterol, osteoarthritis, high vital signs, apnea, and certain sorts of cancer. Public health experts have confirmed the fact that obesity and its health related issues have reached epidemic proportions in this country and around the world.

About a 3rd of U.S. adults are obese. People aged 60 and older are more likely to be obese than younger adults, consistent with the recent data from the National Health and Nutrition Examination Survey. Therefore, the problem also affects children. Approximately 20% of children and adolescents in the U.S. from the age of 2 and 19 are obese.

Who is considered obese?

It is important to understand that to be overweight and to be obese are two different but similar words but differ on a scale that ranges from being underweight to being morbidly obese. Your weight on this scale is determined by your body mass index (BMI). Basically, a BMI is a measure of your weight as it relates to your height. Your BMI gives you a good idea of the amount of body fat you have. Medical healthcare providers use the BMI to find out your risk for obesity-related diseases. It often happens that some muscular people may have a BMI in the overweight range.

However, they cannot be considered overweight because muscle tissue weighs more than fat tissue. In general, adults with a BMI off 20 to 24.9 are considered ideal. A BMI of more than 25 is considered overweight. If a person has a BMI of 30 then he or she is obese, but is considered to have morbid obesity if the BMI is 40 or greater. Generally, the weight of a man above the age of 50 tends to stay the same and often decreases slightly between the age of 60 and 74. But for a woman, this is not exactly the case because a woman's weight tends to increase until age 60 and then begins to decrease.

Obesity can also be measured by waist-to-hip ratio. This particular measurement tool looks at the amount of fat on your waist, compared with the amount of fat on your hips and buttocks. The waist circumference tells the amount of stomach fat. Increased belly fat is associated with type 2 diabetes, high cholesterol, high blood pressure, and heart disease. A waist margin or circumference of more than 40 inches in men and more than 35 inches in women may increase the risk for heart disease and other diseases tied to being overweight.

What causes obesity?

In many ways, obesity is a puzzling disease. Medical Experts have not been able to understand exactly how your body regulates your weight and body fat. But what our common knowledge shows is that a person who eats more calories than he or she uses for energy each day will gain weight. Although, the risk factors that determine obesity can be complicated. This results from the combination of your genes, socioeconomic factors, metabolism, and lifestyle choices. Several medications, disease and health disorders may also affect a person's weight.

Factors that may affect obesity:

Genetics

Generally, recent studies reveal that obesity is passed down through a family's genes. Researchers during the course of study have found several genes that appear to be linked with obesity. Although genes may affect where you store extra fat in your body. However, most researchers think that it takes more than just one gene to cause an obesity epidemic. Further continuous research is crucial to fully understand how genes and lifestyle interact to cause obesity. Your habits, activities and environment also play a major role.

Metabolism factors

Your body utilizes or uses energy differently from how another person does. Hormones and metabolism differ from person to person, and these factors play a role in how much weight you gain. A typical example is ghrelin, the "hunger hormone" that regulates appetite. Researchers have discovered that ghrelin may help trigger hunger. Another hormone called leptin can decrease appetite. Polycystic ovary syndrome (PCOS) is another example, a condition in women caused by high levels of certain hormones. Women with PCOS are more likely to be obese.

Socioeconomic factors

How much income you make may affect whether you are obese. This is especially true for women. More often than not, the poorer or lower status women are more likely to be obese than women of higher socioeconomic status. This is regularly true among minority groups.

Lifestyle choices

Corticosteroids and antidepressants both contribute to obesity. But you can change these lifestyle choices. If your calories come from refined foods or foods high in sugar or fat, you will likely gain weight. If you don't get much exercise, you'll find it hard to lose weight or maintain a healthy weight.

Medicines

Medicines like corticosteroids, antidepressants, and anti seizure medicines can cause you to gain some extra weight.

Emotions

Eating under mental stress or when you're bored or upset–can lead to weight gain. Little or no sleep may also contribute to weight gain. People who sleep less than 5 hours a night are more likely to become obese than people who get 7 to 8 hours of sleep a night.

Health effects of obesity

Obesity has a far-ranging negative effect on health. Obesity-related conditions cost more than $100 billion each year in the U.S and cause premature deaths. The common health effects linked with obesity include;

High blood pressure

An average obese person needs more blood to circulate to the fat tissue and this may cause the blood vessels to become narrow (coronary artery disease). This makes the heart work harder because it must pump more blood against more resistance from the blood vessels which can lead to a heart attack (myocardial infarction). More resistance leads to increased blood circulation which means more pressure on the walls of the arteries. An increased pressure on the walls of the artery will result in a higher blood pressure. Excess weight also raises blood cholesterol and triglyceride levels and lowers HDL ("good") cholesterol levels, adding to the risk of heart disease.

Type 2 diabetes

Type 2 diabetes is majorly caused by obesity. Being obese could make your body resistant to insulin, the hormone that regulates blood sugar. Higher insulin resistance caused by obesity, could drastically increase your blood sugar levels. Even being moderately obese dramatically increases the risk of diabetes.

Heart disease

Overweight or obese people are more prone to atherosclerosis, or hardening of the arteries. The disease of the coronary artery is also more common in obese people because fatty deposits build up in arteries that supply the heart. Arteries that are unevenly narrowed may reduce blood flow to the heart which can cause chest pains called angina or a heart attack. Excess blood clots which form in narrowed arteries and travel to the brain, may cause a stroke.

Joint problems, including osteoarthritis

Obesity can affect the knees and hips because extra weight stresses the joints. An obese person who wants or wishes to undergo a joint replacement surgery may not be a good choice because the artificial joint has a higher risk of loosening and causing more damage. Respiratory problems and sleep apnea are also related to obesity.

Breathing problems for brief periods during sleep are caused by sleep apnea. It interrupts sleep and causes sleepiness during the day. It also causes heavy snoring. High blood pressure is also linked to sleep apnea. Breathing problems tied to obesity occur when the added weight of the chest wall squeezes the lungs. This restricts breathing.

Cancer

It has been stated by the American Cancer Society, that being overweight or obese increases your risk of a variety of cancers.Cancer of the endometrium or the lining of the uterus in younger women is very common among obese women. The chances of Obese women who have gone through menopause having breast cancers are increasingly high. Overweight men have a higher risk of prostate cancer. Obese men and women are at an increased risk of colorectal cancer.

Metabolic syndrome

According to the National Cholesterol Education, metabolic syndrome is a risk factor for cardiovascular disease. Metabolic syndrome has several major risk factors. These factors could be stomach obesity, low HDL cholesterol levels, high blood triglyceride levels, high blood pressure, and insulin resistance (severe type 2 diabetes). These risk factors are common, and having at least 3 of these factors confirms the diagnosis of metabolic syndrome.

Psychosocial effects

Overweight or obese people can have problems psychologically or socially. It is not an uncommon thing that the culture in the U.S. often values an overly thin body image. People that are obese or overweight are often blamed for their condition. Some people may think of them as weak-willed or lazy. It is not unusual for people who are obese or overweight to earn less than other people or to have fewer or no romantic relationships. The disapproval of some people who are biased to those that are overweight may progress to discrimination and even torment. As a result of the constant rejection and discrimination, they usually fall into deep depression.

Chapter 2

The science of food craving

Apparently, food cravings can be pretty complex because they can stem from various mental and physical factors. Oftentimes, food cravings can be triggered by your brain trying to fulfill an emotional need, such as reducing stress and anxiety. During these episodes, three regions of the brain — the hippocampus, insula, and caudate — are all activated almost as intensely as those parts of the brain would in a person with active drug addiction, according to a study published in NeuroImage. Especially, the memory parts of the brain like the hippocampus associate a specific food with a reward that drives these cravings.

Not only the physiological changes, even your lifestyle changes may play a role too. Stress level and chronic lack of sleep or quality rest suppresses a hormone known as leptin that regulates fat storage and calories burned while simultaneously triggering ghrelin, a hormone that causes hunger.

Keeping the body hydrated is important too: if the body doesn't have enough fluids, whether water or otherwise, this can also exacerbate cravings, especially those on the sweeter side. This happens because when your body is not getting enough water it can be difficult for organs that use water such as the liver, to release the food-storing substance known as glycogen or preferably called stored glucose which is a type of sugar obtained from the foods you eat. This then causes your body to crave sweets instead of water.

Why do we crave certain foods?

If you tend to gravitate towards a certain type of food time and time again, there's a reason for that, according to Dr. Berridge. "We crave foods that we're familiar with," he says.

I think it's safe to say that We've probably all craved chocolate and thought to ourselves, "Why can't I crave carrots?" to be honest, it is actually a fair point: Our cravings usually aim for sweet and fatty foods rather than fruits and vegetables.

The truth is, part of it has to do with the fact that these greasier and sweeter foods are tastier and more appetizing. And according to some, biology may be to blame there because in the prehistoric era, our ancestors had to take advantage of these tasty treats where and when they could get them. After all, they weren't as readily available, Dr. Berridge says. That's not the case now — we can easily get them at our nearest grocery store or order delivery from our favorite fast-food restaurant whenever we want.

Though this doesn't happen often, some people even crave non-food items like paper, dirt, or laundry detergent. Dr.

Berridge says this tends to be a sign of a condition called "pica" which could be driven by iron, calcium, or zinc deficiencies.

Should you fight cravings?

Counter to what people might think, you shouldn't fight your cravings. The best way to keep them in check is to acknowledge them, rather than trying to avoid them. "Often, trying to suppress hankerings doesn't work because suppressing means focusing on it, and when we focus on it, we're more likely to give in," Dr. Berridge tells us.

That said, it is still a good idea to come up with a plan for when you start itching for something to eat, especially since we tend to lean toward more fatty and sugary foods.

If you are tempted to indulge, will your cravings be satiated if you do?

Indulging in cravings is not wrong. However, we can understand the concerns if you lean towards greasy or fatty foods and your cravings seem like bottomless pits. Another option is to try to discover more nutritious alternatives to the specific thing you crave.

If you're craving the sugary fruit roll-ups of your youth, you could try dried fruits as a substitute? Other techniques like mindfulness or starting a cravings journal can help you decide when to give in to the urge and when to abstain and identify any potential triggers, like stress or anxiety. Studies have found that your stress levels could drive up your cortisol hormones, which may be linked to hunger, cravings, and compulsive eating behaviors.

The bottom line

Various mental and physical factors cause food cravings. But the good part is that there is rarely a sign that you're lacking the nutrients found in that food. And to get them isn't necessarily negative — after all, they've been key to our survival as humans. "We could not have evolved and succeeded in evolving if we didn't have cravings," Dr. Berridge tells us. "They're what makes us seek food, mates, and other crucial things in life.

Chapter 3

High-calorie diets: the calorie syndrome

Calories obtained from refined, processed carbohydrates has risks. More than two out of every three adults in America are overweight or obese. As stated by the National Health and Nutrition Examination Survey, for some people, this is due to something other than dietary intake such as hormonal disorders. For everyone else, taking in too many calories from foods is the major cause and also not leading an active enough lifestyle. Excess calorie intake not only packs on the pounds but eating too many calories from certain sources causes other health problems. These combined together, can cause an avalanche of issues that negatively impact your overall health and well-being. The good news is that taking charge and making the necessary changes effectively reverses these effects or prevents them from progressing in most cases.

Too many Overall Calories

Weight gain is a major effect of eating too many calories. Calories are needed by your body in specific amounts to function. But when you take in more than your body needs or requires, it stores the excess calories in the form of fat. Excess calories are mainly stored in the form of triglycerides, which when elevated, places your heart health at risk. As with other lipids, too many triglycerides accumulate in your arteries, increasing the risk of your arteries becoming hard, stiff, and narrow -- a condition known as atherosclerosis. The stiffening of the artery walls increases the chances of having a heart attack or stroke.

Once you are overweight, the risk for fatty liver disease, certain cancers, and high blood pressure increases. The increased pressure on your joints raises the risk of osteoarthritis. You could experience breathing problems because of the extra fat surrounding your neck which could lead to sleep apnea, a condition in which you stop breathing temporarily while asleep.

Excess Calories From Carbohydrates

The type of extra calories plays a key role and could affect the health. Too many calories gotten from refined, and processed carbohydrates is common in the U.S. and has its risk factors. Added or extra sugar is a major source of excess calories as a form of refined carbs in the American diet. The health effects of high added sugar intake on insulin sensitivity is still debated. However, consuming too many calories from refined carbohydrates is thought to increase the risk of insulin resistance. A reduced sugar intake significantly improves insulin resistance, according to a study of Latin adolescents in Los Angeles.

The study involved 16-year-old overweight females at the risk of type 2 diabetes. The teens were asked to reduce their sugar intake and increase the amount of whole grains they ate. This slight dietary modification led to better glucose control and lowered their risk of type 2 diabetes, according to the results. The research was published in the Metabolic Syndrome and Related Disorders journal in June 2007.

Excess sugar is a key factor that promotes body inflammation, and atherosclerosis. Excessive sugar intake increases the risk of coronary artery disease, according to an American Heart Association statement published in the journal Circulation in 2002.

Too Many Calories from Saturated Fat

Eating too many calories in the form of trans fat and saturated fat raises the level of total cholesterol in your blood and, in particular, low-density lipoprotein, or LDL -- the harmful form of cholesterol, more so than other dietary components. This matters because elevated levels of LDL are linked to a significantly increased risk of coronary artery disease -- the leading cause of death in the United States. CAD occurs when the main artery that supplies blood to your heart becomes hard and narrow from a buildup of cholesterol. Due to their structural characteristics, LDL promotes atherosclerosis more than other types of fat.

Reducing Calorie Intake

Make a conscious effort of reducing the amount of calories you take in if you know you're eating too much. These little changes can have a big impact on your health risks. You could Completely try to avoid trans fats, and replace some saturated fats with unsaturated fats. The best sources of unsaturated fats include oily fish, nuts and seeds, and plant-based oils like olive and sesame.

Substitute added sugars with sweet whole foods such as fruit. The amount of sugar found in fruits is naturally low, and because fruit contains fiber, it reduces the rate at which sugar enters your bloodstream, making it a much healthier choice of sweet food.

If you're like most Americans, and you're not getting enough servings of fruit each day, you could take fruits with you on the go as a snack, or keep fruits available in bowls at home. Because added sugar is the major source of added calories in a typical diet, it's a good place to start. You can also start cutting back because it has the beneficial result of lowering your overall calorie intake. Focus yourself on making healthier food choices, and you'll reap the health benefits.

Chapter 4

The potential of fitness: how regular exercising can transform your life

Regular exercising has a lot of benefits, resistance training can help with weight loss by maintaining muscle mass and boosting metabolism. Cardio could also be helpful but may make you hungrier, so try to eat mindfully.

If you're trying to lose weight, you may be wondering how much you should be exercising and what types of exercise you should be doing. In the simplest way, losing weight means burning more calories than you consume. So, it makes sense to include exercise in your routine, since it helps you burn more calories.

However, strenuous exercise can also help you work up an appetite. This may confuse the role of exercise in weight loss and whether it can help. So, you may ask yourself, what exactly is the purpose of exercise if you're trying to lose weight? This book takes a look at the evidence to help you find the answer and figure out what's best for you.

Cardio exercise and weight

One of the most popular types of exercise for weight loss is aerobic exercise, also known as cardio: are;
walking
running
cycling
swimming

Aerobic exercise may not have a major effect on your muscle mass, at least not compared to lifting weights. However, it is a highly effective way of burning calories. A 10-month study examined how cardio without dieting affected 141 people who were obese or overweight. Participants were split into three groups and not told to reduce their calorie intake

Those who burned 400 calories per cardio session (5 times per week) lost 4.3% of their body weight, while those who burned 600 calories per session (also 5 times per week) lost a little more, at 5.7%. The control group, which didn't exercise, actually gained 0.5% of their body weight. Different studies also show that cardio can help you burn fat, especially the dangerous belly fat that increases your risk of type 2 diabetes and heart disease. This means adding cardio to your lifestyle is likely to help you manage your weight and also improve your metabolic health if you keep your caloric intake the same.

However, resistance training — such as weight lifting — has other benefits that go way beyond that. Resistance training helps increase the strength, tone, and amount of muscle you have. One study of 141 older obese adults examined the effects of cardio, resistance training, or both on body composition during a period of intentional weight loss. And the result of the study found that those who did no exercise or cardio alone lost fat but also lost more muscle and bone mass than the groups that did resistance training. So, it can be said that resistance training appears to have a protective effect on both the muscles and the bones during periods of reduced calorie intake.

A higher muscle mass also increases your metabolism rate, helping you burn more calories. Around the clock — even at rest. This is because muscles are more metabolically active than fat, meaning it requires more energy. This also helps in preventing the drop in metabolism that can occur alongside weight loss.

Because of this, doing some form of resistance training is a crucial addition to an effective long-term weight loss plan. Keeping the weight off is easier, which is much harder than losing it in the first place. Lifting weights helps to tone, maintain body shape, build muscle and it helps prevent your metabolism from slowing down when you lose fat.

High-intensity interval training and weight

High-intensity interval training (HIIT) in simple terms, is a type of exercise characterized by short bursts of intense exercise followed by a brief rest before repeating this cycle. HIIT could also be done with cardio or resistance training exercises and provides the benefits of both.

Most HIIT workouts are only 10–20 minutes long, but they offer some powerful benefits regarding weight loss. A 2017 review of 13 high-quality studies found that HIIT and cardio exercise provided similar benefits — namely, reduced body fat and waist circumference — for people that are overweight and Obese.

However, HIIT exercise achieved these same benefits with a 40% time saving compared to cardio. Due to the intensity of HIIT, it is advisable you consult a healthcare professional before starting a new HIIT routine, especially if you have known heart concerns.

Exercise and appetite

We've all probably heard that physical exertion is a good way to work up an appetite, or maybe you even found yourself eating more than usual after a vigorous workout. However, some studies point to exercise having an appetite suppression effect.

A study of 20 active and healthy adults noted that they ate more food in the meal before a workout than after — and actually found that the overall participants ate less food on the days they exercised than on the days they didn't. In another study with 26 women who were obese on low-calorie diets, researchers found that short HIIT sessions had a significantly strong appetite-suppressing effect.

Researchers have also noted that exercise done in the morning appears to be more beneficial for energy balance and calorie intake than evening exercise — further supporting the theory that exercise can reduce appetite.

Regardless, more conclusive research is needed, and hunger responses to exercise are likely highly individual. If you tend to eat more than usual while trying to lose weight, or after vigorous or long exercise sessions, consider shorter durations (like HIIT) or less intense exercise.   A regular exercise could make you more or less hungry; however, research mostly points to exercise having an appetite-reducing effect.

Other benefits of exercise

Exercise and its benefits cannot be understated because, it is really great for your health in many ways, not just in terms of weight management. Effective exercising can improve your blood sugar control and may help reduce your risk of chronic diseases like heart disease, type 2 diabetes, and certain cancers.

Exercising is helpful in growing and maintaining your muscle mass, keeping your bones strong and dense, and to prevent the onset of conditions like osteoporosis — which is characterized by bone brittleness.

Additionally, exercise offers some mental benefits. It not only helps you by reducing your stress levels and managing stress more effectively, it appears to offer some protection against neurodegenerative conditions like Alzheimer's disease.

Keep these benefits in mind when you're considering the effects of exercise. Even if it doesn't make a huge difference in weight loss, it still has other benefits that are just as (if not more) important.

Chapter 5

Maintaining energy balance

What you consume is a major component when it comes to energy and weight loss, but there are other natural factors you can implement in your journey to ensure you stay active for longer.

Start small

When you first embark on your weight loss path, it can be tempting to make drastic changes instantly. However, this could set you up for failure as you and your body could get thrown into the deep end without having time to adjust. If you want to ensure the longevity of your new lifestyle change, then start small and slowly switch out bad foods and go easy at the gym – this will ensure your mood and hormones stay in check.

Exercise

Keeping yourself active is a great way to boost energy. You may not realize it but partaking in that 40-minute jog on the running machine, or even getting some fresh air and going on a walk with a friend can get your heart rate up and get the blood to flow which in return releases endorphins and raises energy levels. Instead of wandering to the sofa to binge-watch your favorite series, wander outside instead (you can thank us later).

Sleep

As humans, we need to recharge. Getting less amount of sleep each night can lead to us feeling exhausted and unhappy the next day…and the days to come. Reducing your calories and also switching up your usual routine can add added stress to your body, so it's crucial to make sure you give your body the rest it needs – Sleeping for about 7 to 9 hours is perfect to be precise.

Schedule meals

With dieting it may be easy to fall into the routine of skipping meals, especially with a busy schedule, but this will have no benefit to you whatsoever. Eating meals at regular intervals throughout the day can help manage blood sugar as well as stabilize your mood. Try not to go longer than 4 hours between meals and snacks – it's time to begin meal prepping!

Keep hydrated

The role water plays in weight loss is crucial because dehydration can make an individual feel irritable, tired, and ill. You are also more likely to wreck your diet as dehydration can cause hunger pains which makes your body conclude that instead of water, it needs food to handle the low energy. So, make sure your water bottle is filled up at all times.

Factors in a treat

Completely limiting yourself off all your favorite naughty snacks can wreak havoc on your mental health and in return affect your energy levels. The simple fact is, consuming these salty and sugary treats day in and day out won't do anyone any good, but factoring in a KitKat or a packet of salt & vinegar Walker crisps every so often is a great idea to make sure you look forward to something. Keep your mindset in tip-top position. After all, it's much better to have a cheat meal than a cheat day.

Embracing a new weight loss routine whilst boosting up your energy levels is challenging for most. Your body takes time to adjust, and it's always worth noting that things don't happen overnight (we wish they did). Knowing the right kind of food to eat and the regime to take is vital - we hope that we have helped to make your life that much easier, as well as providing that extra bit of motivation. So keep Staying positive and keep up the good work, we believe in you.

Conclusion

" The concept of Obesity " offers an innovative and creative perspective on obesity, shedding light on the science behind food cravings, metabolism, and sustainable weight loss. It provides a wealth of evidence-based information, empowering readers to take charge of their health and make informed choices to beat obesity's challenges. This comprehensive guide may be a valuable resource for anyone seeking to scale back, improve energy levels, and embrace a healthier lifestyle.